# Meal Plan

By: Wannabe Balanced Mom
Crystal Escobar

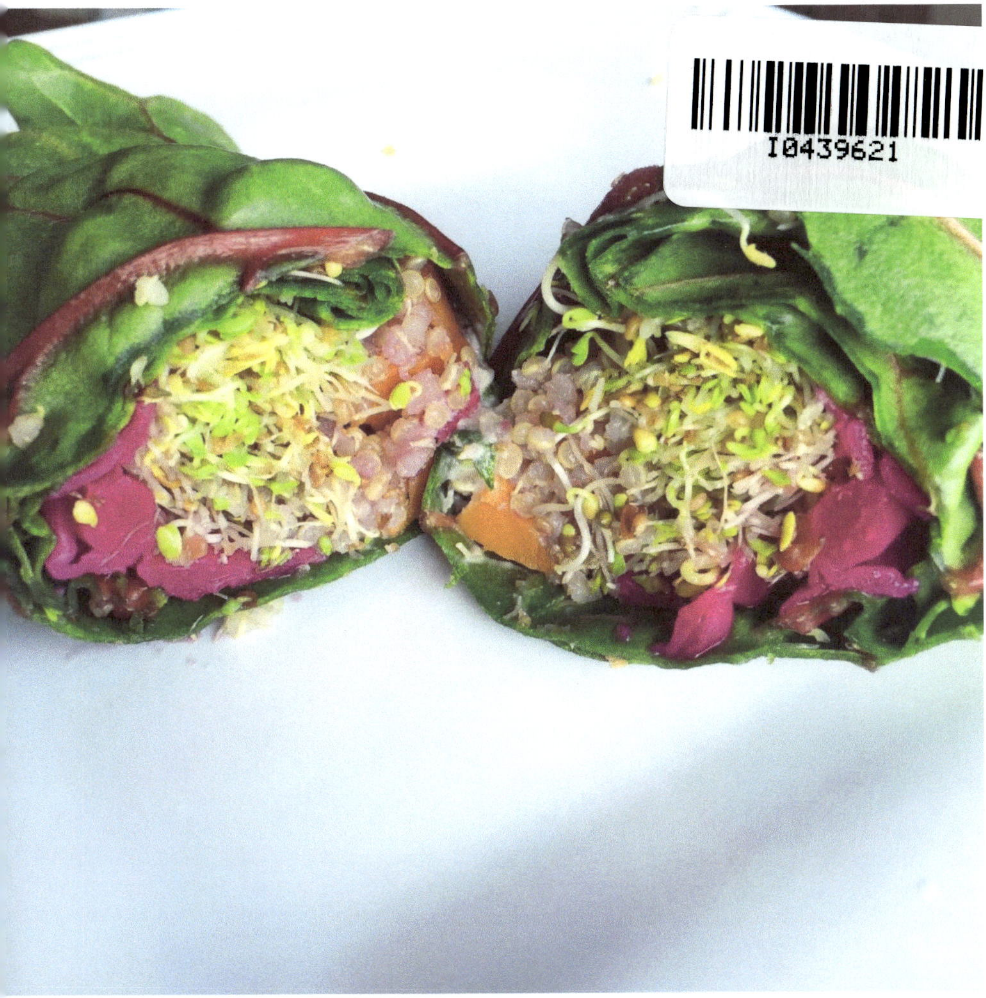

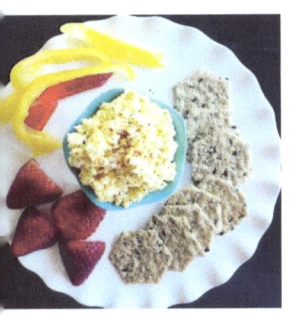
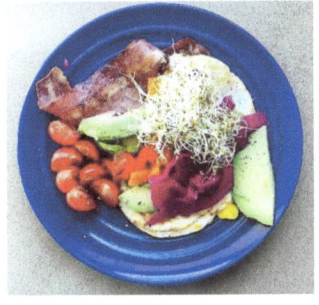
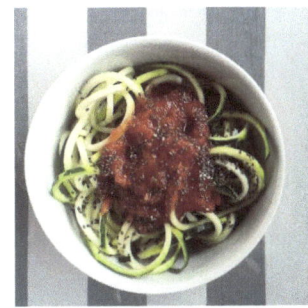

## Stay Connected:

Instagram: @CrystalEscobar2
Facebook: @Wannabe Balanced Mom
Blog: www.WannabeBalanced.com
Periscope: @CrystalEscobar
Text: 801-792-9759
Email: crystal@escoweb.net
Request More info: www.wannabelean.com

# Getting Started

It's very important that you take the time for some meal prepping. I like to do it on Saturdays because that's the day my husband is available to help with the kids. A lot of my meals include fermented veggies and kefir, so if you're not familiar with that then I encourage you to get my printable PDF with all the instructions needed.

### STEP 1
Grocery shopping. Take a picture, screen shot, or print out the grocery list I've provided, then head off to the grocery store.

### STEP 2
Wash all your fruits and veggies, then chop and store in separate containers.

### STEP 3
Make your Quinoa
Bake your sweet potatoes
Soak some walnuts
Start sprouting your lentils
Start sprouting the Buckwheat groats
Grill some chicken if you plan to use it

### STEP 4
To make everything else run smoothly this week I encourage you to make some of the foods that can be stored in the freezer, like the avocado ice cream, brownies, and protein pancakes.

I've tried to organize the meal plan in such a way that will require minimal prep each day. I ALWAYS double my recipes because I like to have extras to freeze for quick meals on a different day. So you will need to decide how much you should make with each recipe provided. It all depends on whether or not your husband and children will be eating these meals with you.

Although this meal plan is only for one week, keep in mind that this ONE week meal plan can be your blue print for many months to come. It's simple to mix things up a little but still sticking with the same guidelines. For example, experiment with different beans when making your sprouted patties. Or use different greens in your salad or for the veggie wrap, use different toppings on your gluten free pizza, use different nuts or seeds, make spaghetti squash instead of zoodles, healthy cookies or muffins instead of brownies, make a banana peanut butter ice cream instead of avocado ice cream (just frozen bananas, a little almond milk and peanut butter or PB2), ect. Everything can be mixed up as long as you stay within the category the food belongs to.

My healthy eating habits have definitely evolved over the years. I didn't just wake up one day and decide I was going to eat a mostly vegan and gluten free diet. It's happened over the course of 10 years, little by little finding healthy alternatives to the foods and drinks I love. Kombucha has become my Diet Coke, Kefir has become my yogurt, my protein shakes have become my ice cream, zoodles are my new pasta, and gluten free brownies give me my chocolate fix.

One thing you must keep in mind, is that it's OKAY to fall off your meal plan. Don't beat yourself up over it, just try again NOW! Don't wait until tomorrow, this moment right now can be a fresh start. So you gave into your cravings and ate a big hamburger with french fries and a milk shake. It's OKAY! Eating clean does not happen over night, it's a process, something to get used to, so take it little by little and never give up.

Some of my recipes call for cultured foods because I'm a firm believer of the importance of probiotic foods in your daily diet. But if you've not experimented with fermented foods yet then no worries. Just substitute fresh veggies for the cultured veggies, or yogurt for the Kefir. If you DO want to learn more about how to make these then you can purchase my PDF instructions for $3.

# GROCERY LIST

## Produce:
Spinach
Avocados
Romaine lettuce
Other lettuce of choice
Choose a leafy green veggie
like kale, swiss chard, ect.
Sweet potatoes
Berries (lots of berries)
Cherry tomatoes
Red cabbage
Bell peppers
Zucchini for zoodles)
Toppings for pizza (you decide
what you like)
Asparagus
limes
Sprouts

## Fish & Poultry:
Chicken breast
fish of choice (I like Tilapia or
Salmon)
Turkey bacon
Eggs and or egg whites

## Dairy:
Kefir, yogurt, or cottage cheese

## Sweetener:
(You don't need all of these,
just choose 3)
Stevia
Coconut sugar
Agave
Date sugar
Honey

## Nuts & Grains:
Pine nuts
Walnuts
Quinoa
Granola
Lentils
Steel cut oats
Regular oat meal
Chick peas
Buckwheat groats
Pumpkin seeds
Chia seeds
Ground Flaxseed
Almond meal
Gluten free flour blend (or
make your own with brown
rice flour and tapioca flour)

## Frozen:
Berries

## Other:
Protein shake
Brown rice cakes
Quinoa
Peanut butter
PB2
Chocolate covered hemp or
chia seeds (find on Amazon)
Marinara sauce
Green drink powder
Cocoa powder
Arrowroot powder
Coconut oil
Non diary chocolate chips
Almond milk
Coconut milk in the can
Gluten free crackers
Italian seasoning
Mexican seasoning

# Weekly Blue Print

## Monday

**Breakfast:** Isalean Shake (pg.10)
**Snack:** Rice cake with peanut butter and chocolate covered hemp seeds. (pg.12)
**Lunch:** Spinach quinoa salad with sweet potatoes, avocados, and cultured cabbage. (pg.13)
**Snack:** Avocado Ice Cream (pg. 14)
**Dinner:** 2 sprouted patties with kefir cheese and cultured bell peppers (pg.15)

## Tuesday

**Breakfast:** Granola with fresh fruit and almond milk (pg. 16)
**Snack:** Protein shake
**Lunch:** Quinoa with asparagus, fresh tomatoes and pine nuts (Pg. 17)
**Snack:** Kefir smoothie (pg. 18)
**Dinner:** Taco lettuce wraps (pg. 19)

## Wednesday

**Breakfast:** Buckwheat bowl (pg.20)
**Snack:** Rice cake with peanut butter and chocolate covered chia or hemp seeds.
**Lunch:** Salad with sprouted patties (pg. 21)
**Snack:** Protein pudding (pg. 22)
**Dinner:** Gluten free pizza (pg. 23)

# Thursday

**Breakfast:** Protein shake
**Snack:** Egg with turkey bacon, avocado and sprouts (pg.24)
**Lunch:** Left over gluten free pizza
**Snack:** Healthy brownie (pg.25)
**Dinner:** Fish with left over asparagus and sweet potatoes (pg.26)

# Friday

**Breakfast:** Kefir with fruit and sprouted buckwheat groats(pg.27)
**Snack:** Protein shake
**Lunch:** Taco salad with left over taco meat(pg.28)
**Snack:** Avocado ice cream
**Dinner:** Spag. squash or zoodles (zucchini noodles) with marinara sauce (pg.29)

# Saturday

**Breakfast:** Protein shake
**Snack:** BLT (pg.30)
**Lunch:** Protein pancakes (pg.31)
**Snack:** Oatmeal with fruit and coconut whip cream (pg.32)
**Dinner:** Veggie wrap with sprouts, avocados, cultured cabbage (pg.33)

# Sunday

**Breakfast:** Protein pancakes
**Snack:** shake
**Lunch:** Salad with everything on it (pg.34)
**Snack:** Healthy brownie
**Dinner:** Kefir green smoothie/ gluten free crackers or chips with guacamole, hummus, or egg salad (pg.35)

I want to explain to you just how amazing the IsaLean protein shakes are and how they compare to all others on the market. This shake is actually THE most important meal in this whole plan because of the quality and perfectly balanced and top quality ingredients.

I gained almost 50 lbs with each one of my pregnancies and have been able to lose it all every time, thanks to my healthy lifestyle that includes, cleansing and the daily consumption of perfectly balanced meals in shake form. I have been drinking these delicious shakes for over 11 years now and believe me when I say that these shakes are the #1 most important piece to my weight loss success. Of course I believe that cleansing is also very important, but I'm most passionate about daily nutrition and how that can affect your weight and health overall.

Most of us are busy moms and finding time to create healthy nutritious meals each day is extremely tough. That's why I love that I can replace at least one meal a day with these no brainer meals. One less thing to worry about right? I don't believe in fast food, but this is the only exception. With only 240 calories, its the perfect nutrient-dense food.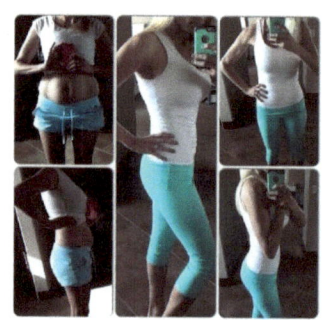

Now I'm fully aware that Shakeology and Isagenix are going head to head in competition as far as the amount of consumers go. So let me break down the difference between these two shakes. It's important that you do your research and look into the ingredient sources.

Is Shakeology a good shake? Yes. Does it beat the IsaLean? No! Here's why-

## Protein~

"The whey protein isolate in Shakeology shakes is denatured! Unfortunately, nearly every single whey protein supplement out there is denatured. Fortunately, Isagenix isn't one of them, which I'll explain in a second.

When talking about whey protein and how it's processed or created, not all processes and whey proteins are created equally. Whey is the byproduct of cheese making. Most companies use salts, enzymes, acids or heat to separate out the curds from the whey and casein. These 4 processes absolutely change whey and casein. This type is called "denatured" meaning the proteins are altered through chemical or physical means so that some of its original properties are lost or diminished.

There's another way in which the curds and whey and casein can be separated. It's a patented, exclusive process called cold, ion exchange micro-filtration. This process does not use the above-mentioned 4 processes. This process is how our Isagenix undenatured whey protein concentrate, milk protein concentrate and low-heat non-fat dry milk is created. This process is incredibly expensive but protects the whey in its natural God-given state, protecting all the dipeptides and tripeptides, yielding an amazing amino acid profile too.

These undenatured proteins are then cold air dried in a huge spray-drying drum, using no heat and then the proteins are carefully sealed in crates. Our whey comes from New Zealand, free-range cows that are grass fed (free from herbicides, pesticides etc.), milked and rested according to season and free of hormones, antibiotics and steroids. These are happy cows. This whey is exclusive to Isagenix!"

*source~ Shakeyourwaytosuccess*

## COST~

"Not only is IsaLean and Greens more affordable but each serving yields 24 grams of undenatured protein vs. Shakeology's 17 grams of denatured protein. With Isagenix, you're getting better quality period. "

*Source~ Shakeyourwaytosuccess*

| Product | Cost- 30 servings | Cost per meal | Calories | Grams of Protein |
|---|---|---|---|---|
| Isagenix IsaLean plus Greens | $110 (39+39+32) | $3.66 | 240 | 24 |
| Shakeology Chocolate | $119.95 | $4.00 | 140 | 17 |

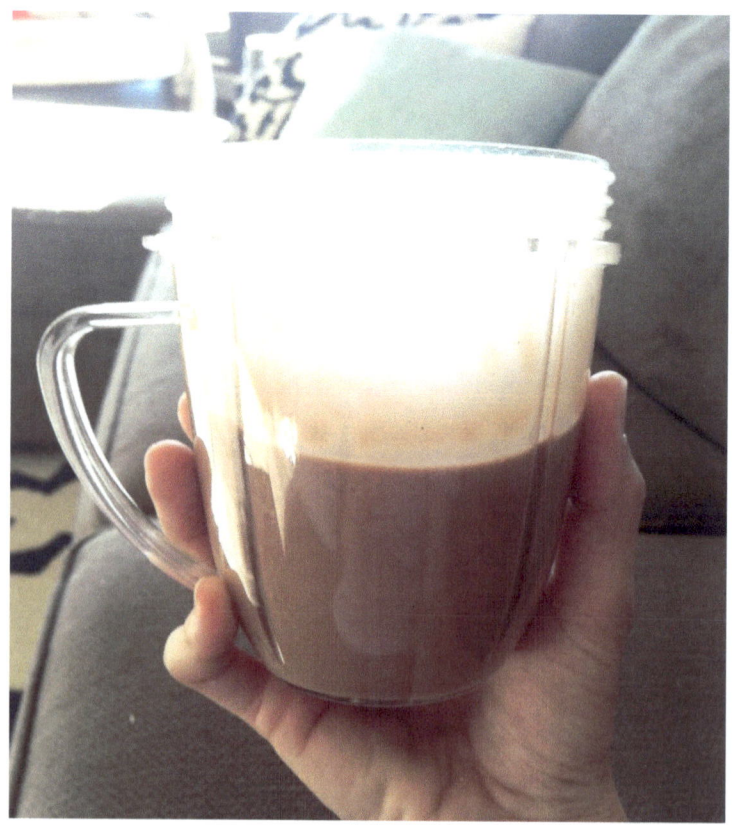

What makes IsaLean Shake superior?

IsaLean is a full meal replacement—not a "snack," providing optimal support for nutritional cleansing and replenishing, weight loss and weight maintenance, as well as peak performance. While low in saturated

fat, sodium and cholesterol, IsaLean® Shake provides the right balance of protein, carbohydrates, healthy poly- and mono-unsaturated fats, dietary fiber, vitamins and minerals (including calcium, vitamin C, vitamin B12, and vitamin D). Plus, you get active digestive enzymes that help maximize absorption of key nutrients. Many products touted as "meal replacements" don't deliver adequate nutrition to do the job of replacing a meal. Plus, most don't have the right amount of protein to prevent the muscle loss that often accompanies weight loss. IsaLean Shakes need only to be blended with water for a satisfying meal replacement while many others require being mixed with milk in order to even come close to being a proper meal replacement.

Below is a short testimonial and before and after picture I thought was a perfect example of how quality can really make a difference in results. I found this information on Trueglutenfree.com

The before picture of us below was after doing 3 months of P90X3 and drinking Shakeology for 6 months. The after picture, was literally 2 weeks later and the ONLY thing that changed in my diet or day-to-day routine was that we stopped taking Shakeology and started on an Isagenix 30 Day Nutritional Cleansing System.

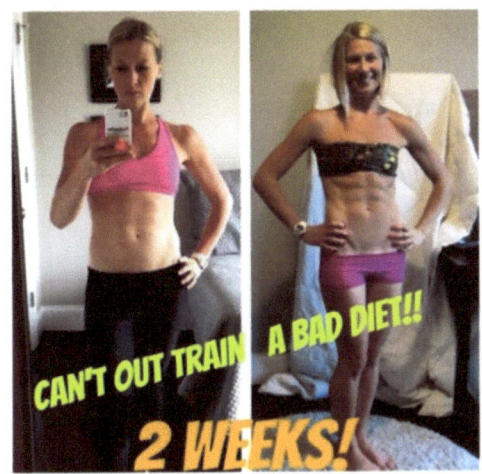

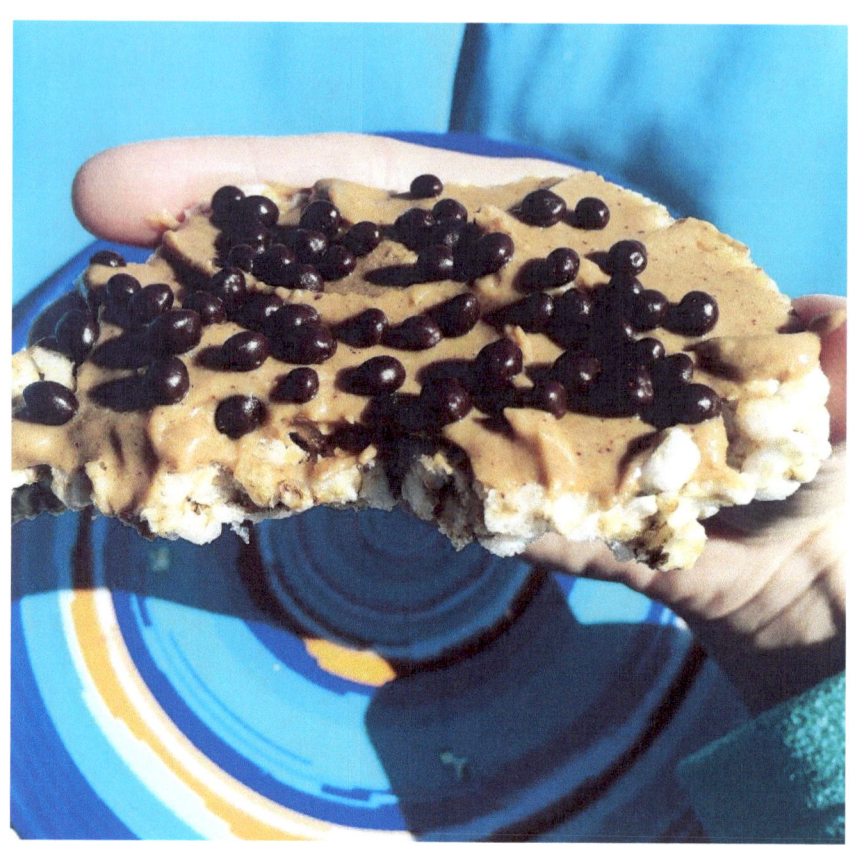

Okay, this snack/treat is amazing! Ever since I bought these chocolate covered hemp seeds, I've been putting them on everything! My two year old thinks they are Nerds candy. This brown rice cake topped with peanut butter and chocolate covered hemp seeds is the perfect snack or treat. (You can find these chocolate covered hemp seeds on Amazon, they even have chia seeds).

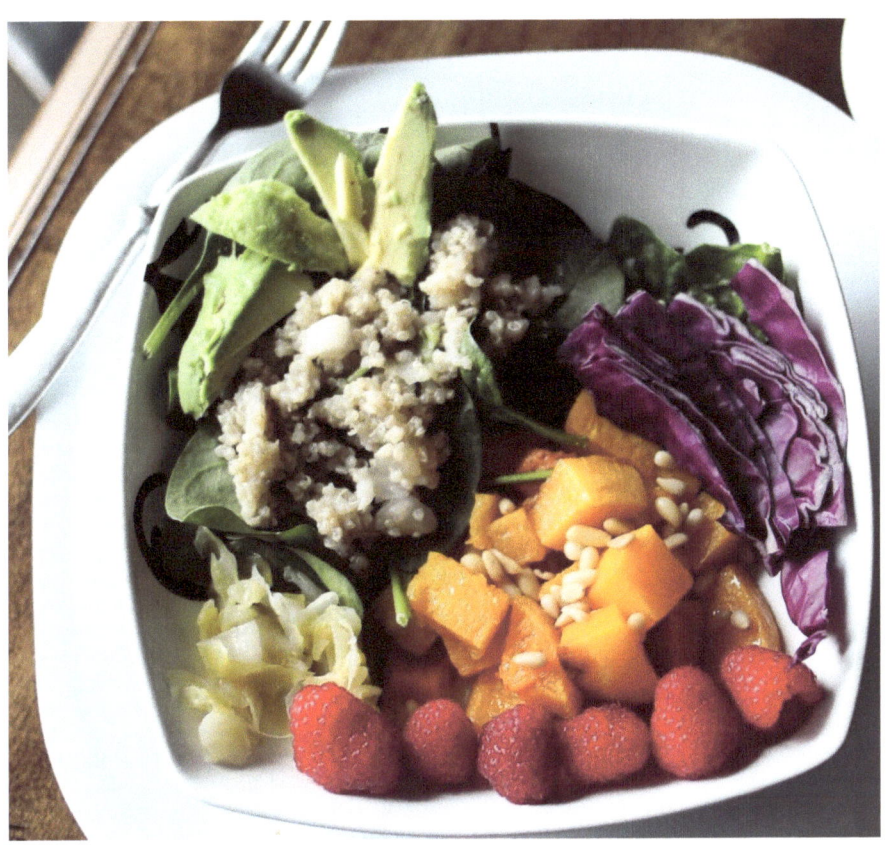

I love getting creative with salads and adding lots of color. Choose a green, doesn't have to be spinach. You can use kale, or romaine lettuce too. Just top with some cooked quinoa (with coconut oil and salt in it), avocados, baked sweet potatoes, pine nuts, purple cabbage, with a side of cultured cabbage. I try to add a couple table spoons of cultured veggies to every meal because it helps with the digestion of raw foods. Then use a healthy dressing of choice. I like to just drizzle a little olive oil and vinegar on top then sprinkle different herbs or seasonings.

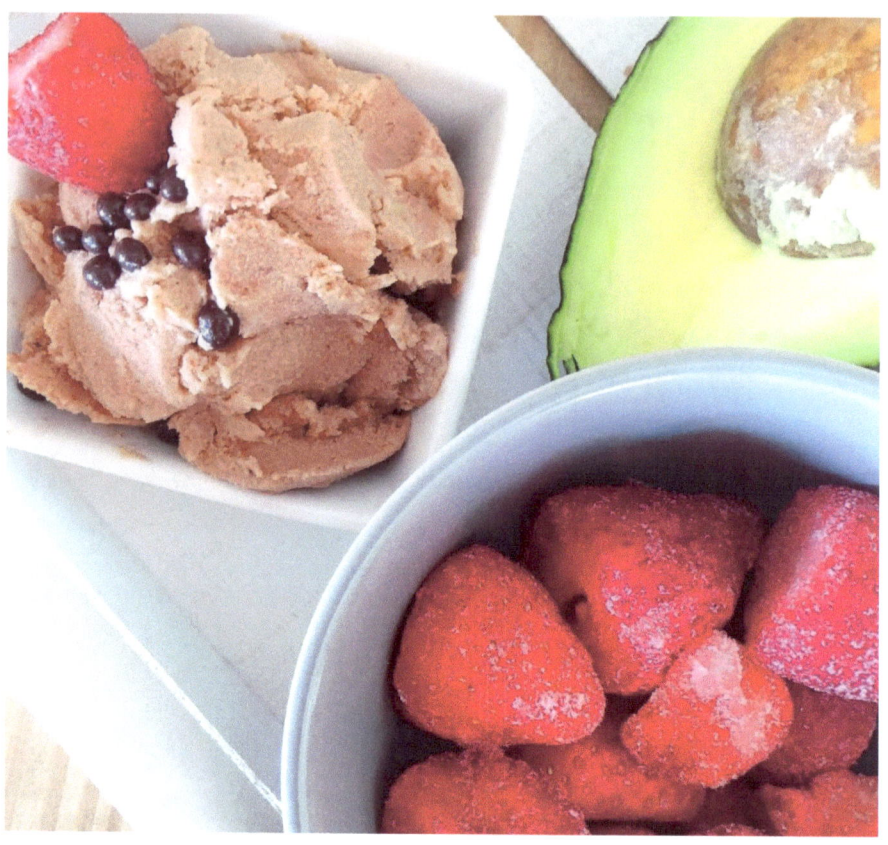

## Avocado Ice Cream

Here is a delicious dairy free ice cream with lots of omegas and protein. My two year old LOVES this stuff and I'm so excited about it because I've never been able to get my kids to eat avocados. All you do is add 3 avocados and 3 cups frozen strawberries with 3 T agave and 1 tsp. vanilla extract. You'll have plenty left over for your family or to eat on another day. Just store in an airtight container in the freezer. Get creative with the toppings. Of course you know how much I love the chocolate covered chia seeds and hemp seeds, but I also love to sprinkle crushed home made graham crackers on top. You can also find healthier graham cracker, or cookie options at the health food store. Just make sure you just sprinkle a little on, don't go overboard with the toppings if you want to lose weight. Try to keep your meals at about 200-300 calories.

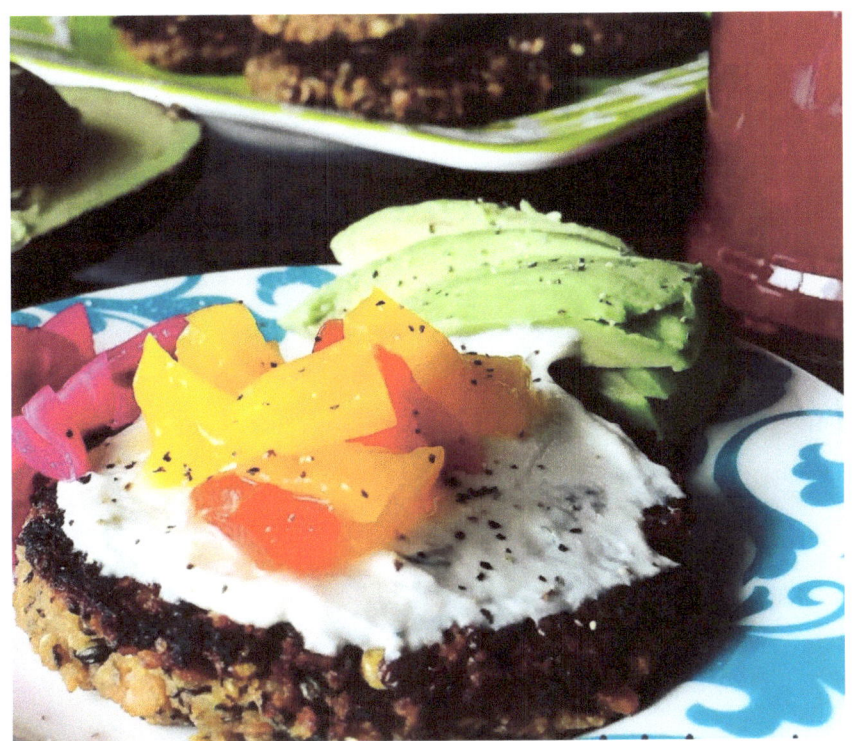

## Sprouted Patties

Blend two and a 1/2 cups of sprouted lentils (you can also use
Garbonzo beans or any other kind of bean) with about 1/4 cup
tomato sauce, 1/4 tsp garlic powder (or 3 fresh garlic cloves), 1/2 tsp
salt, 1/4 tsp pepper, other seasonings of choice and one tsp. of gluten
free flour (I used brown rice four).

Heat some coconut oil in a skillet, then spoon the mixer into the pan
(use the spoon to flatten and shape into patties). Cook until golden
brown and flip.

## KEFIR CHEESE TOPPING:

Make kefir cheese by placing a colander in a bowl. Place a coffee
filter in the colander, then pour the kefir into the filter and let sit in
the fridge for a few hours but for best results let sit overnight. This
process will remove the liquid whey from the kefir creating a nice
thick sour cream like consistency.

Then once you have your kefir cheese just add a little fresh dill,
garlic powder and salt. AMAZING I TELL YA!!!!

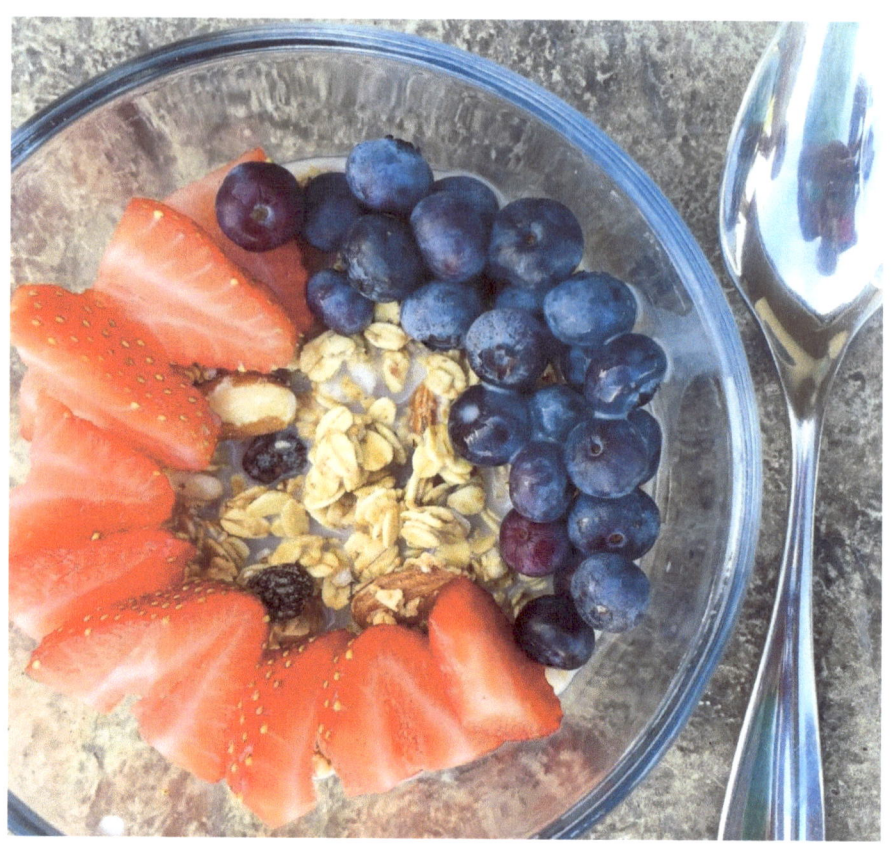

## Granola with almond milk and berries

If you'd like to be extra ambitious then I'd recommend
making your own granola. This way you have control over
what goes in it and the amount of sugar content. To be
honest, I have not gotten around to making my own YET, but
I will be doing it very soon. In this picture I'm using an
organic brand I bought at Harmons. I just chose the one with
the least amount of sugar content.

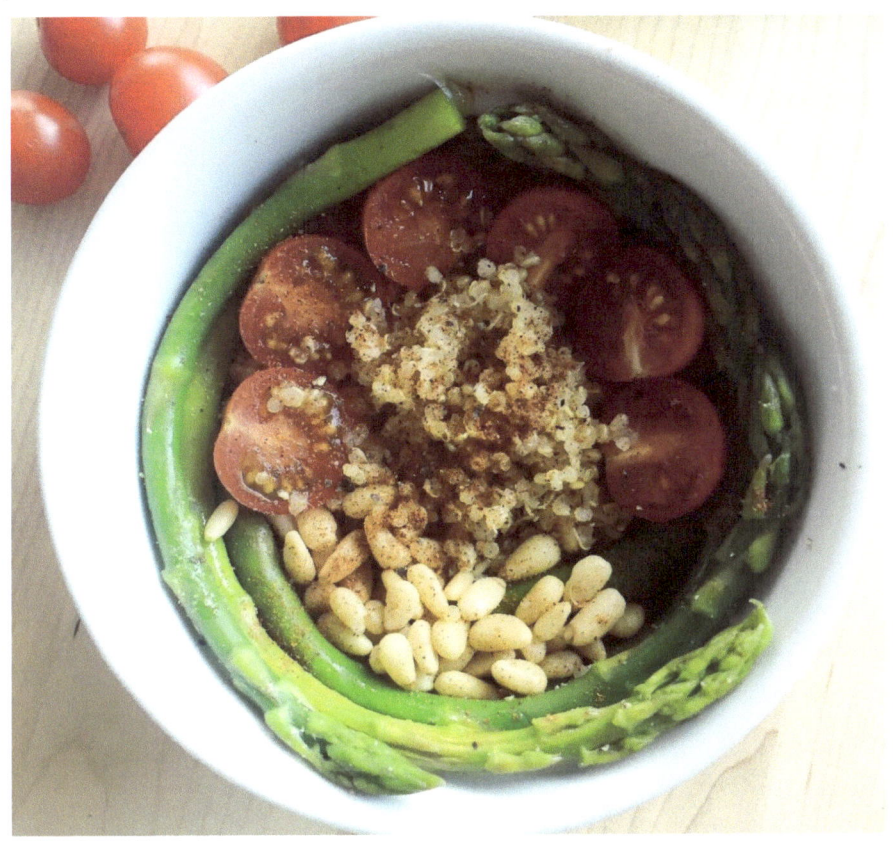

### Quinoa Asparagus Bowl

Beautiful and simple bowl of goodness. Just used quinoa that was cooked in Organic Better Than Bouillon (chicken base). Streamed asparagus seasoned with lemon pepper, fresh cherry tomatoes, and pine nuts, sprinkled with a little salt and pepper. Get creative and add some other spices like garlic or chili powder, YUM!

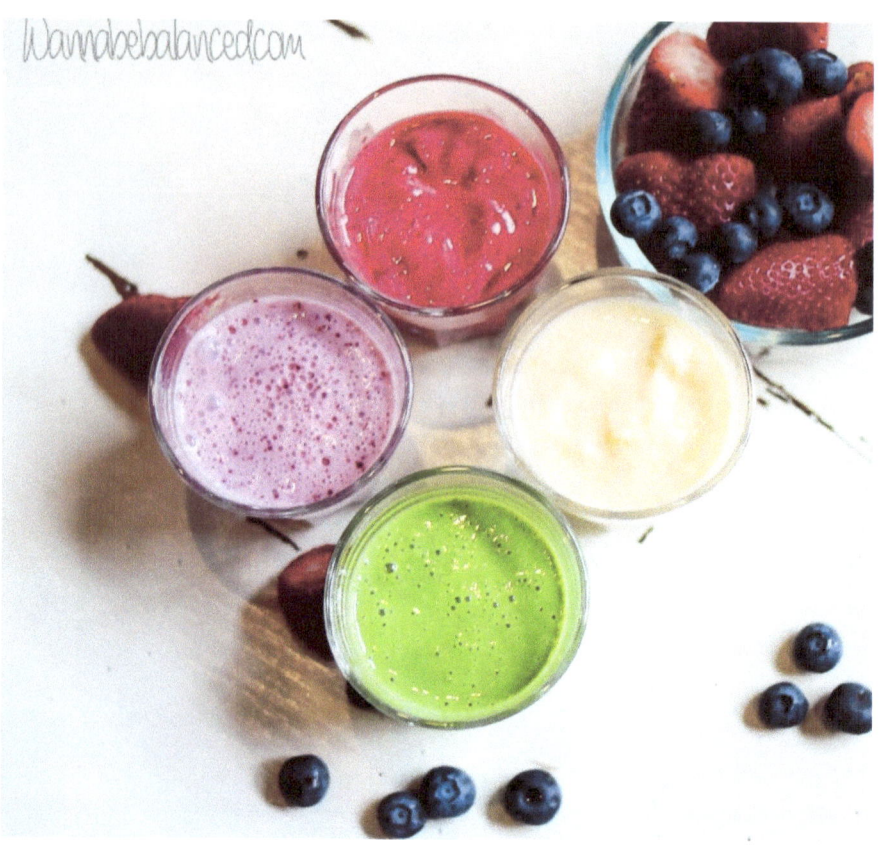

## Kefir Smoothie

You all know that I'm a firm believer in making your own Kefir. First of all, it's super simple, and second of all, it's packed full of probiotics and and has no lactose OR sugar because of the fermentation process. Usually yogurt from the store is packed full of sugar, and most yogurts are pasteurized, which means that most of the enzymes and healthy bacteria have been killed off. Kefir has 30-56 strains of good bacteria and store bought yogurt only has 10.
In your kefir smoothie all you need to do is add 2 cups kefir and 2 cups fruit mixed with spinach. May favorite is 1 cup frozen strawberries, 1/2 banana and a huge handful of spinach. You can even drizzle a little vanilla extract and sprinkle some cinnamon for added yumminess.

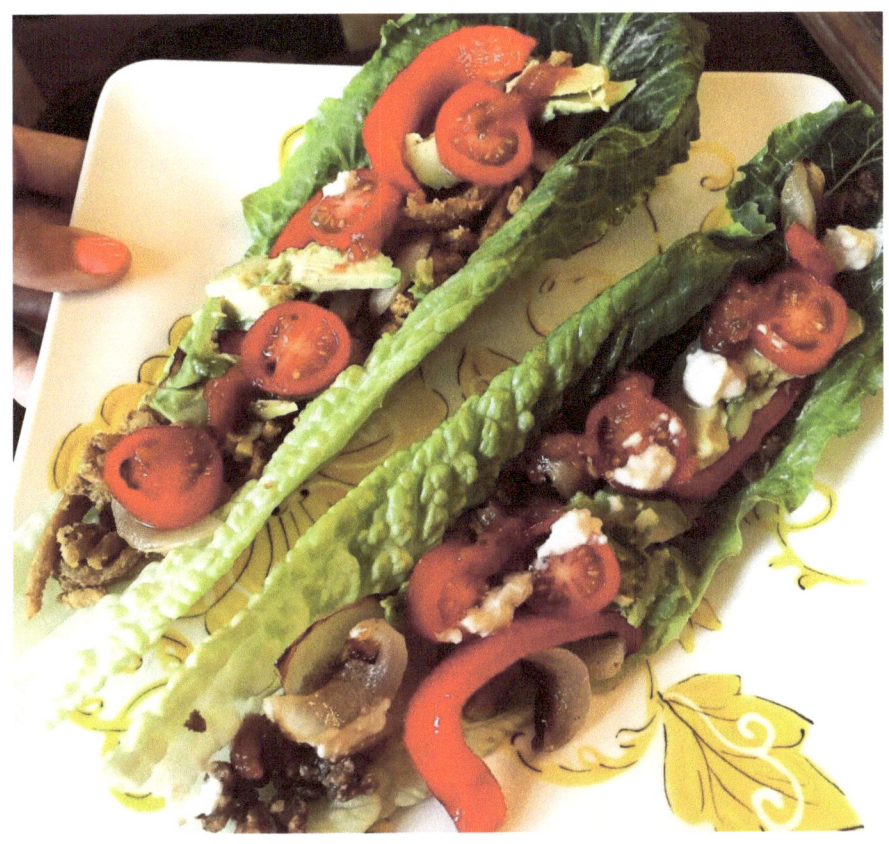

## Taco Lettuce Wraps

Two options here. I like to eat a mostly vegan diet, but if you can't do it then go ahead and substitute the walnut "meat" with ground turkey meat. Basically all you do to make the walnut meat is, soak 2 cups walnuts in water for two hours, or over night in the fridge. Then in a food processor, add walnuts, and 2 T of Mexican seasoning ( I make my own in large batches, but for this recipe it's just 1 T cumin, 1 T coriander, dash of garlic powder, dash of paprika, and dash of black pepper and salt.) 2 T balsamic vinegar, and 1 T olive oil. Pulse several times until crumbly, making sure not to over blend. Spread the taco meat on the lettuce leaves and garnish with grilled peppers and onions, avocado, and cherry tomatoes. Squeeze fresh lime juice over the top then sprinkle with a little more salt and pepper.

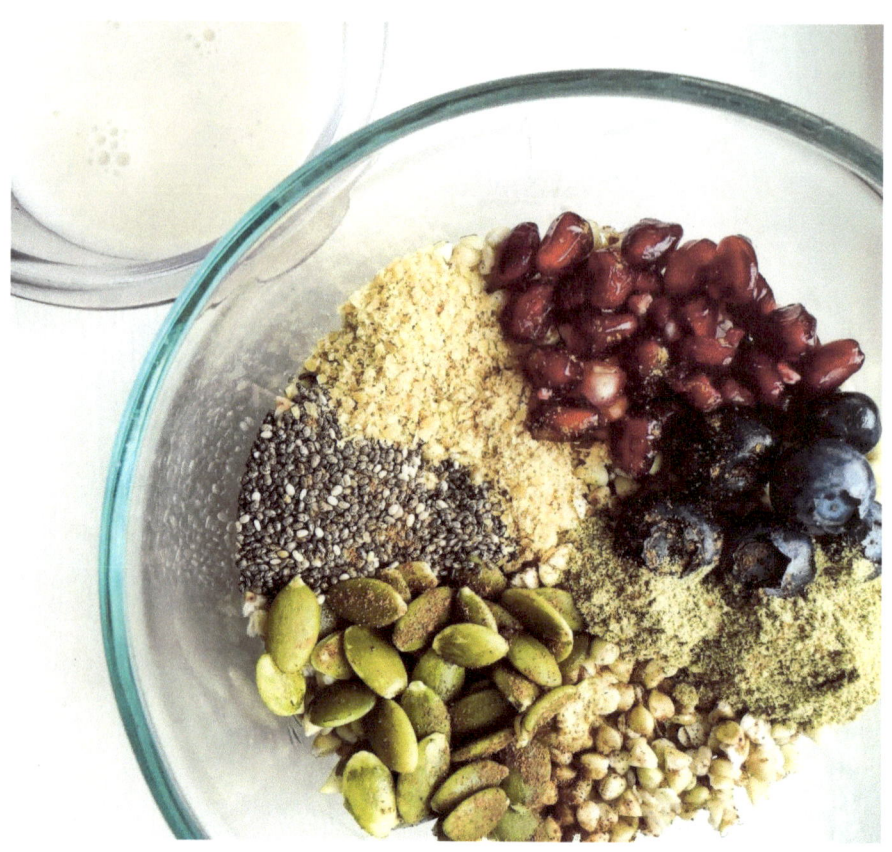

### Buckwheat Bowl

Raw sprouted buckwheat with ground flaxseed, chia seeds, pumpkin seeds, fresh berries, healthy greens powder (I use the Isagenix brand), sprinkle of cinnamon and a little almond milk. You eat it just like cereal and it is 100 times more nutritious than any kind of cereal you can find at the store.

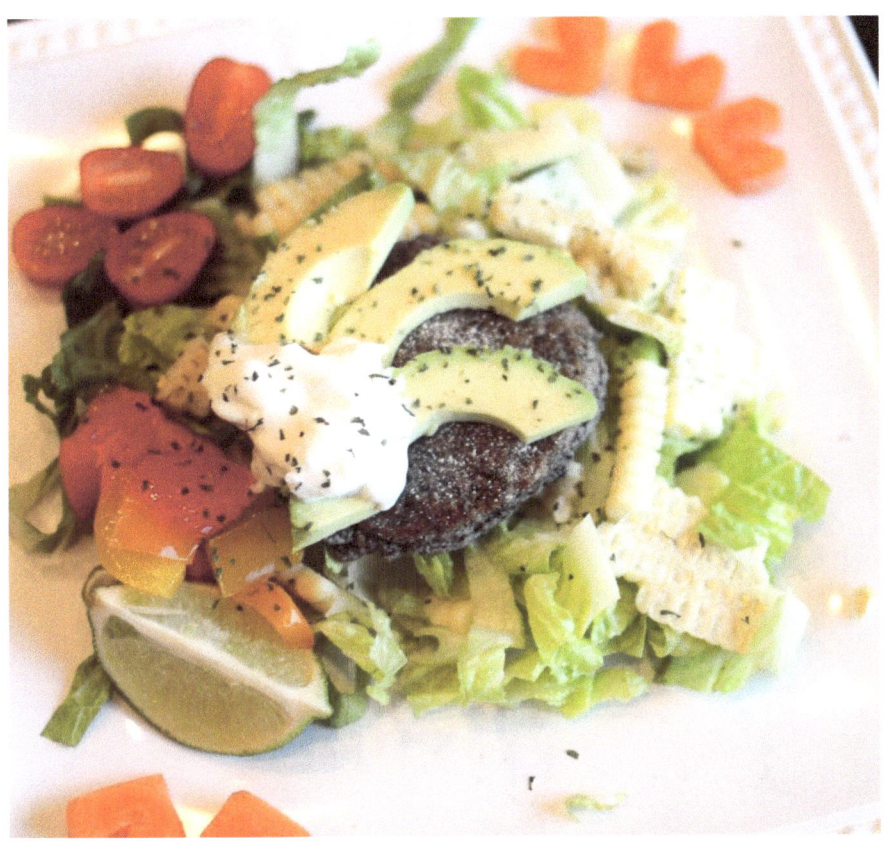

## Salad w/sprouted bean or lentil patty

The fun thing about these sprouted patties is that you can get creative with it. Just choose your bean or grain, sprout them, then blend it up with different seasonings. This one in the picture is a sprouted black bean patty with mexican seasoning. Now just add it to a nice green salad, throw in some fermented veggies, kefir cheese, avocados and tada! You have a beautiful salad with a wide variety of nutrition. Another thing I love about these patties is that you can make a bunch of them and pop in the fridge of freezer for a simple ready to go meal for another day.  Just place them in the toaster for a quick reheat.

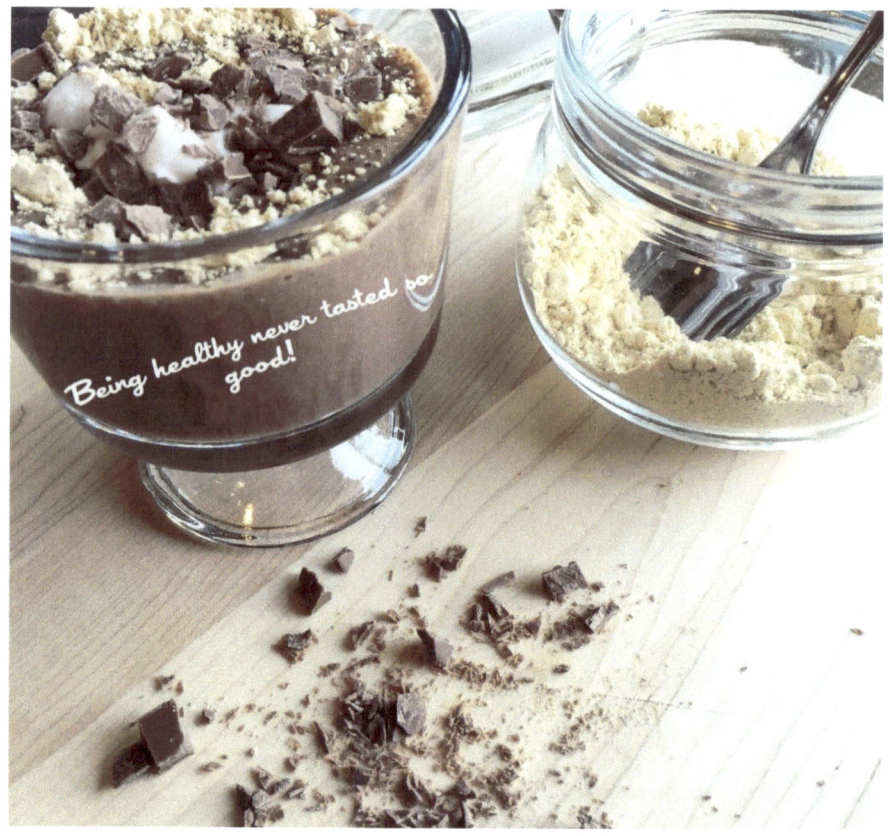

### Protein Pudding

It's so fun to get creative with your protein shakes. One of my favorite ways to make my shake more like a dessert is simply add only 1/2 cup of water with some ice or a small piece of frozen banana, blend it up then sprinkle some PB2 and chocolate chunks on top. Even better, place it in your freezer for about 30 min. before eating. I'm addicted to the chilled pudding like texture.

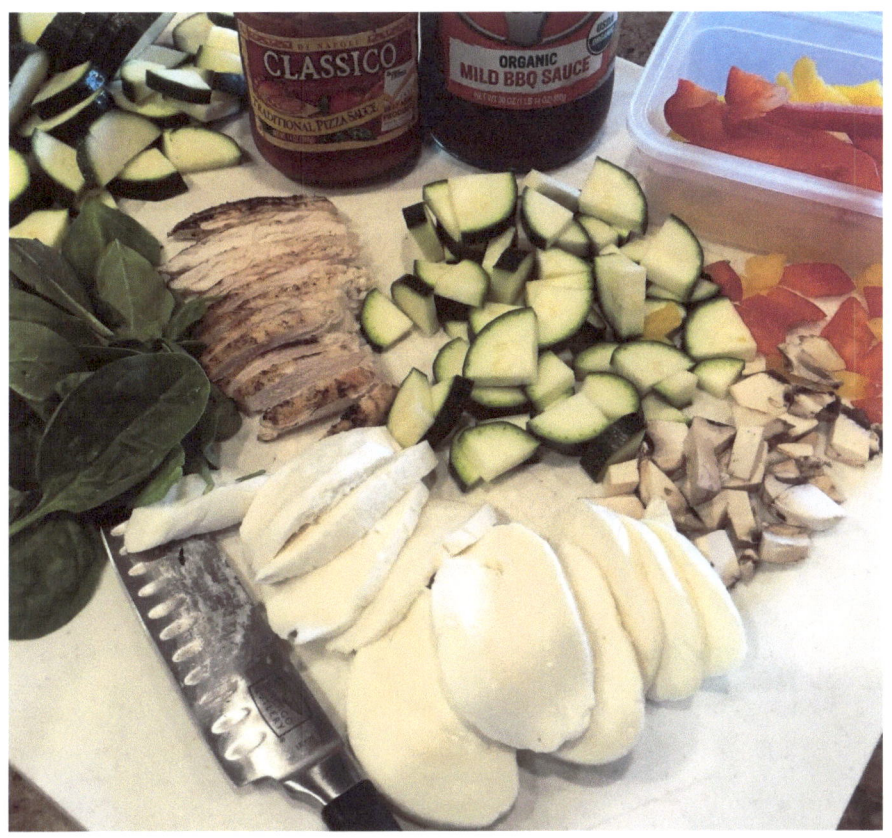

## Gluten Free Pizza

I'm in love with this gluten free pizza. If you can find I nice GF flour blend then your pizza will turn out nice and chewy. Heat oven to 450 degrees F. Spray baking sheet with non stick spray or just rub on some coconut oil. Then just combine 2 1/2 cups GF flour blend (brown rice flour, tapioca flour, and a little Arrowroot flour is a nice combo). Then 1 1/4 cup water, 1 tsp garlic powder, 1 tsp baking powder or Arrowroot, some Italian seasonings,  and 1 T coconut oil. The consistency will be kind of gooey so what I usually do is cover my hands in coconut oil then use my hands to flatten out the dough onto a baking sheet to create the crust. Bake for about 20 minutes on lowest rack. Pull the crust out and add sauce and toppings. then bake an additional 10-15 minutes. Save left over pizza because you will be eating it tomorrow for lunch.

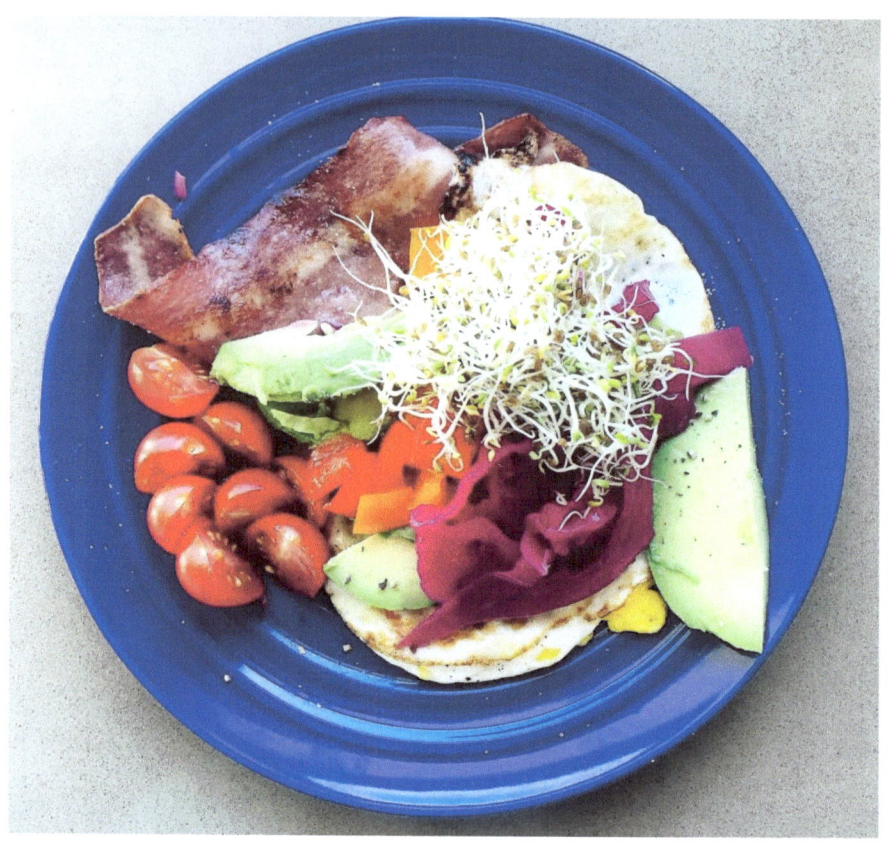

### Turkey Bacon Egg Avocado

If you were diligent in your meal prep then you should have your fermented foods and sprouts on hand at all times. This dish is loaded with goodness and should only take you 5 minutes to prepare. One slice of turkey bacon, one egg, 1/2 avocado, a few cherry tomatoes, fermented red cabbage and some sprouts. As you can see I love to add as much color and nutrition to every meal.

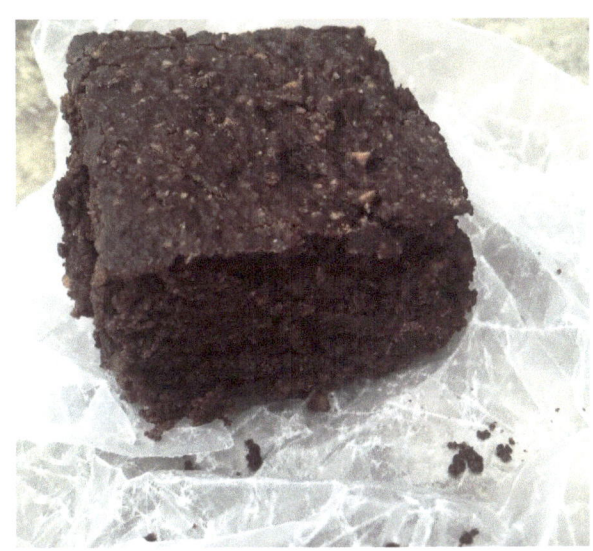

## Vegan GF Brownies

Although I'm obviously not vegan, I do however eat a mostly vegan diet. I believe our bodies need some animal protein for optimal health. So here is my favorite brownie recipe inspired by Oh She Glows.

Ingredients:
- 2 T ground flax + 3 tbsp water, whisked
- 3/4 cup + 2 tbsp brown rice flour
- 1 cup  almond meal
- 1/2 cup cocoa powder
- 2 T Arrowroot powder
- 1/2 tsp sea salt
- 1/4 tsp baking soda
- 1/4 cup + 2 tbsp Coconut oil
- 1/2 cup cup non-dairy chocolate chips
- 1/2 cup agave
- 1/2 coconut palm sugar
- + 1/4 cup date sugar or stevia
- 1/2 cup almond milk
- 1 tsp vanilla
- 1/2 cup finely chopped walnuts

- 1. Preheat oven to 350F. Line a 9 inch square pan with parchment and grease all sides. In a small bowl, whisk together the ground flax and water and set aside.
- 2. In a large bowl, whisk together the dry ingredients (flours, arrowroot, cocoa, salt, baking soda).
- 3.  Add in flax liquid, sugar and agave, vanilla, coconut oil, and almond milk. Whisk.
- 4. Pour wet mixture over dry mixture and stir well. The mixture will be VERY dry, but not to worry keep mixing! Now fold in the walnuts chocolate chips.
- 5. Scoop thick batter into prepared pan
- 6. Bake for 35-37 minutes at 350F and allow brownies to cool in pan

25

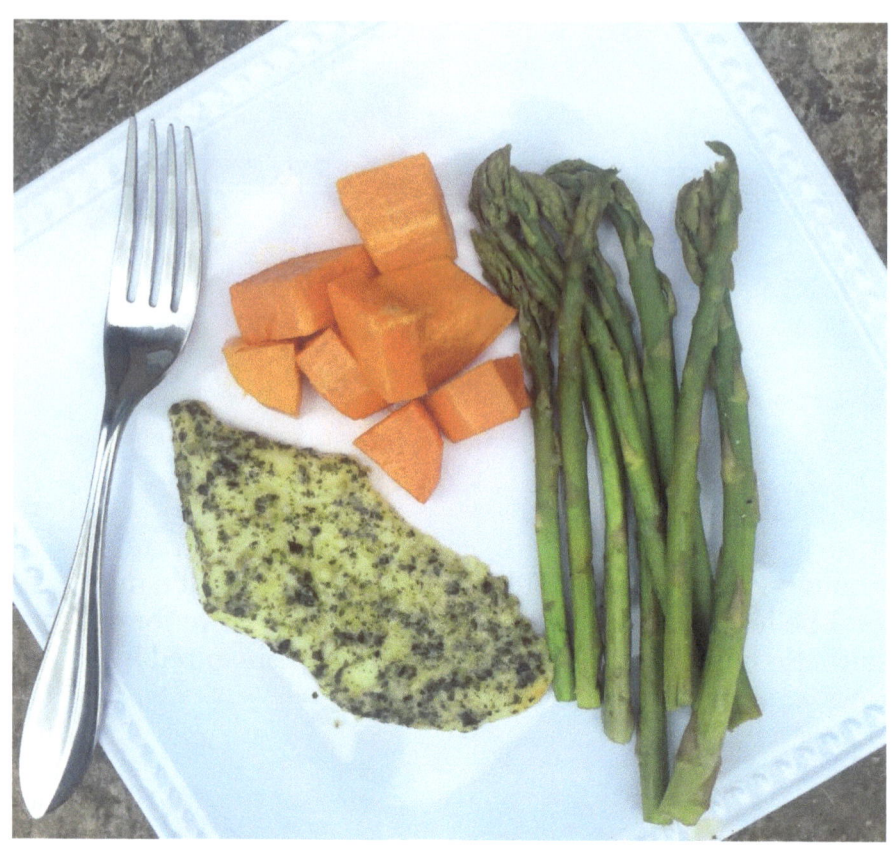

### Fish w/Sweet Potatoes & Asparagus

I love buying the already seasoned fish from Costco. Our favorite is the Tilapia and Salmon. This meal is super simple since you've already baked your sweet potatoes earlier this week. Now just pop the fish in the oven and steam your asparagus. After you steam your asparagus just drizzle a little olive oil and sprinkle some lemon pepper on top.

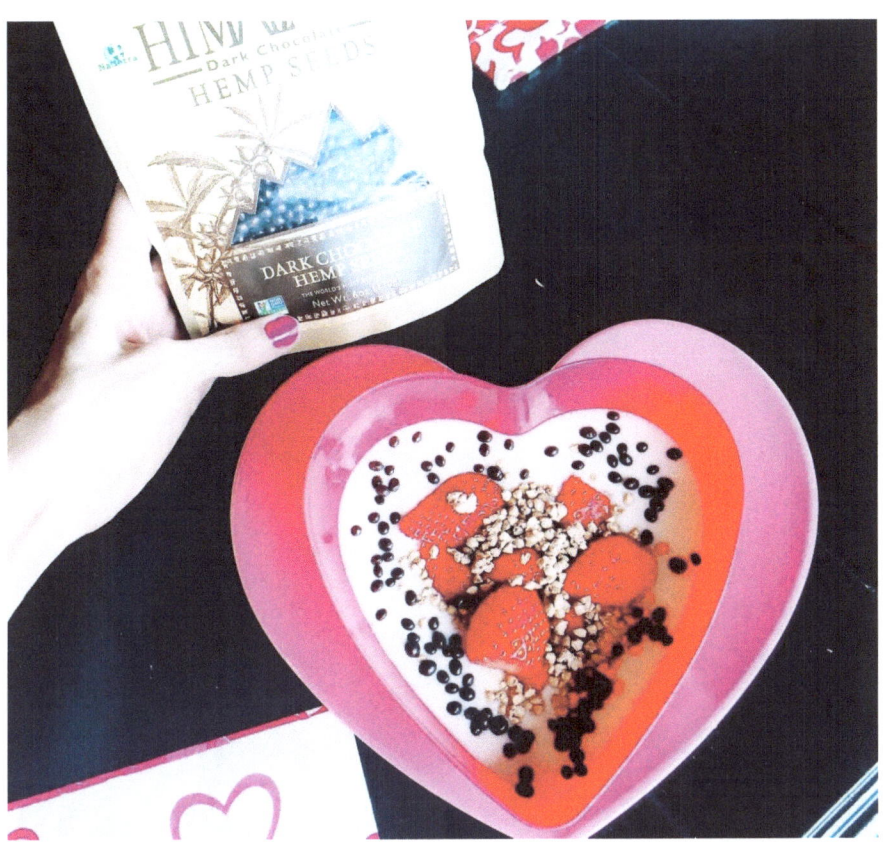

## Kefir w/Fruit & Buckwheat

Kefir is also great as a yogurt bowl replacement. Just add a little stevia to sweeten it, fresh berries, sprouted buckwheat groats and sprinkle some yummy chocolate covered hemp or chia seeds on top.

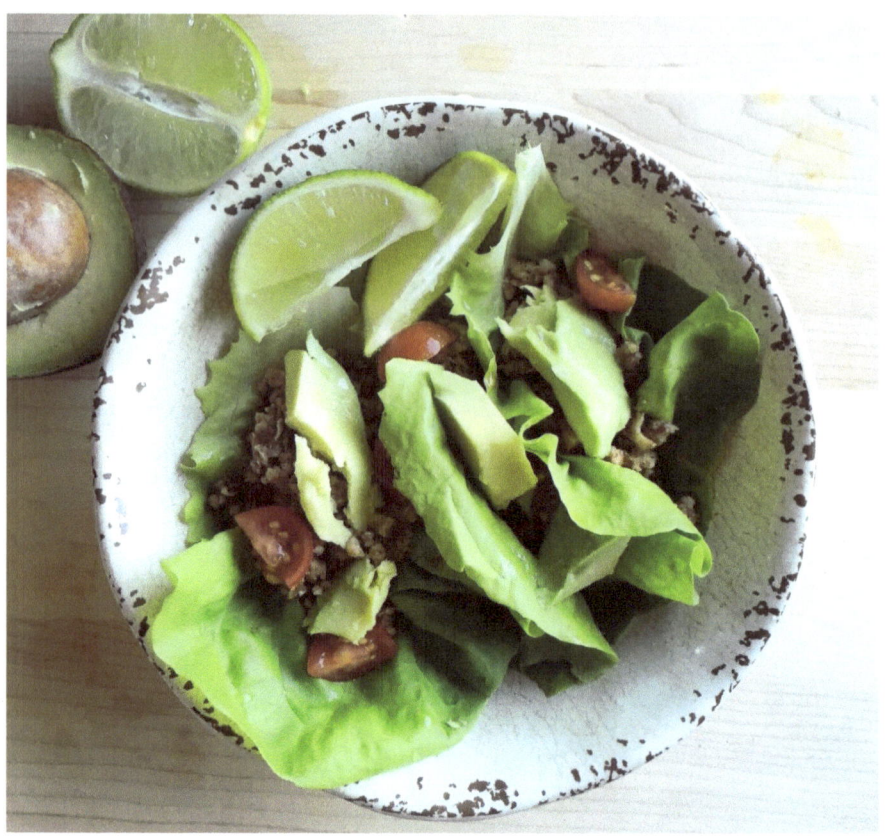

### Vegan Taco Salad

I love making good use of my meal prep time, so I ALWAYS make extra when making anything. This saves me so much time. Now that I already have my vegan taco "meat" already prepared, all I have to do is throw a little lettuce in a bowl, add some tomatoes and avocados then drizzle on a little dressing of choice.

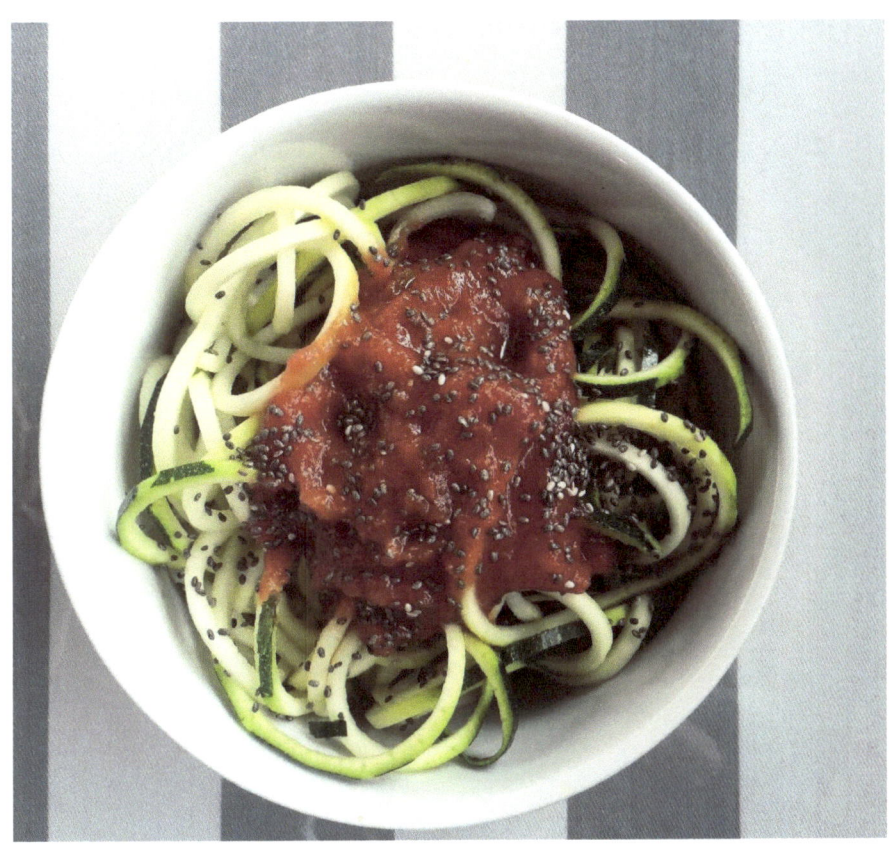

### Zoodles w/Marinara sauce

If you don't have a zoodle maker then no worries, you can do spaghetti squash or even just chop up the zucchini into little pieces. Then just put the zucchini and sauce into a pan with a little coconut oil. Heat it up but don't really cook it. So literally just a few minutes in the pan. This way you won't lose much of the nutrition AND the zucchini won't get all mushy.

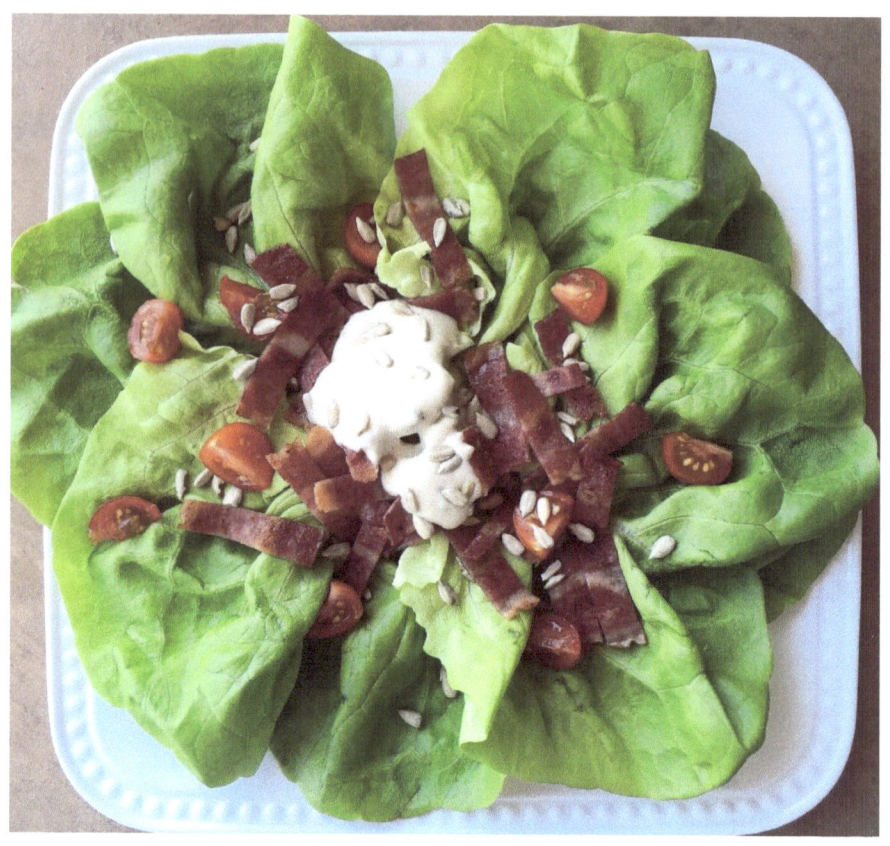

## BLT

Isn't turkey bacon the best? Gives every dish so much flavor! This salad will literally take minutes to put together. If you've done your due diligence on meal prep day then your lettuce should be all washed and ready to go. Then cook up the bacon, add your tomatoes, sprinkle some sunflower seeds, and add a dollop of Kefir cheese (with ranch seasoning) and you're done!

*If you don't have kefir then use a dairy free ranch dressing.

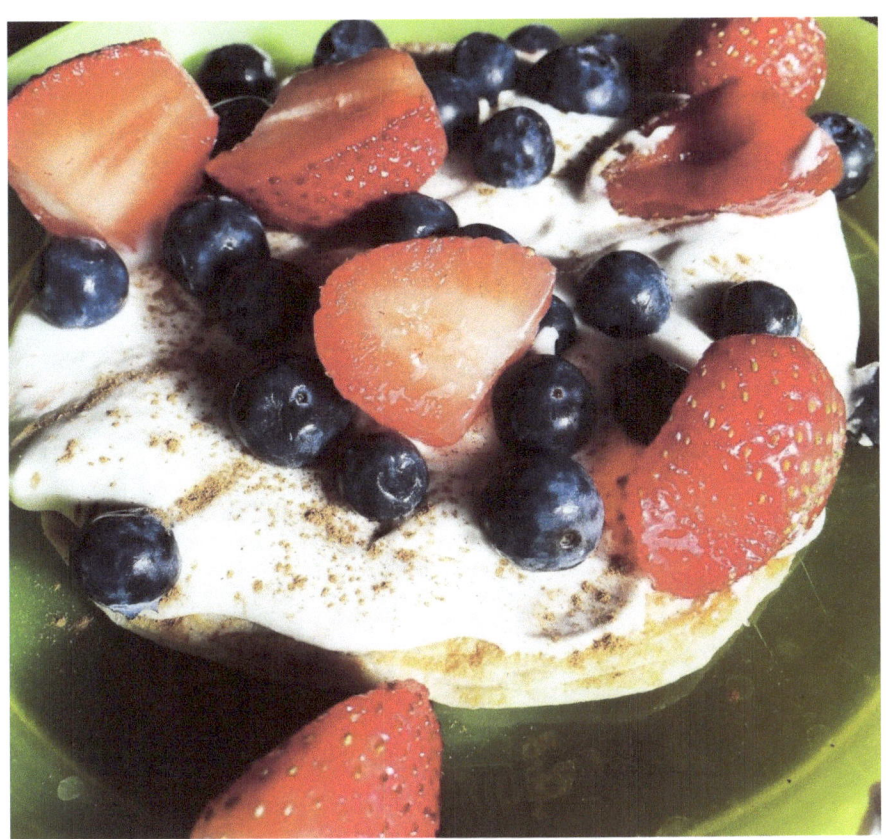

## Protein Pancakes

Protein pancakes is one of my favorite go to because you can make a huge batch and freeze them for an easy nutritious snack for another day. I like to top mine with vegan whip cream, berries and a sprinkle of cinnamon. You can also do almond butter as a topping which is amazing. So to make these pancakes, all you need to do is add 2 cups oatmeal flour (blend oatmeal in a vitamix to create the flour), 2 cups Kefir (or blended cottage cheese, or Greek yogurt), 2 cups egg whites (or 8 eggs), 2 scoops of vanilla protein powder. Mix it all together and now you have your batter. Just coat your pan with a little coconut oil and cook like regular pancakes. I highly recommend doubling this recipe and just making a ton all at once. These are so nice to have on hand.

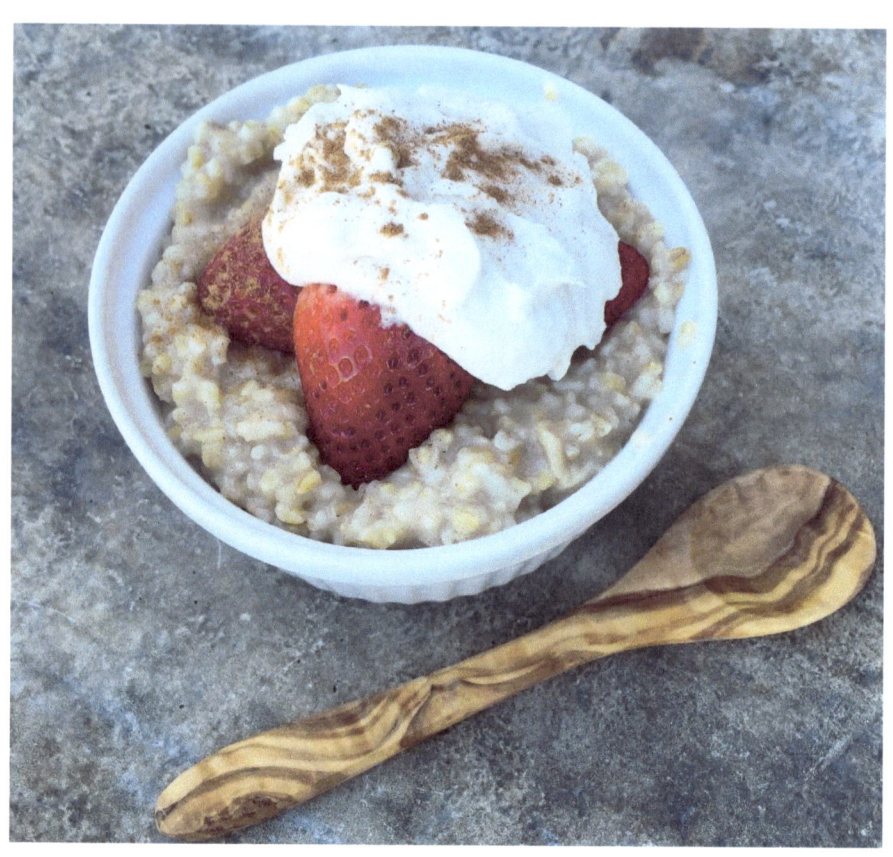

## Oatmeal Bowl

Oatmeal is such a beautiful thing right? You can get so creative with this stuff, add all different kinds of fruit, coconut whip cream, seeds, nuts, spices, and even a little protein powder if you're trying to get more protein in. This is one of my favorite snacks but it feels like a treat. I usually have steel cut oats because I love the chewy texture, then I add a little coconut oil, stevia, and some 100% maple syrup to sweeten. Also, I do love to add a little vanilla protein powder and some seeds to this bowl. I just forgot to add the seeds before I took this picture.

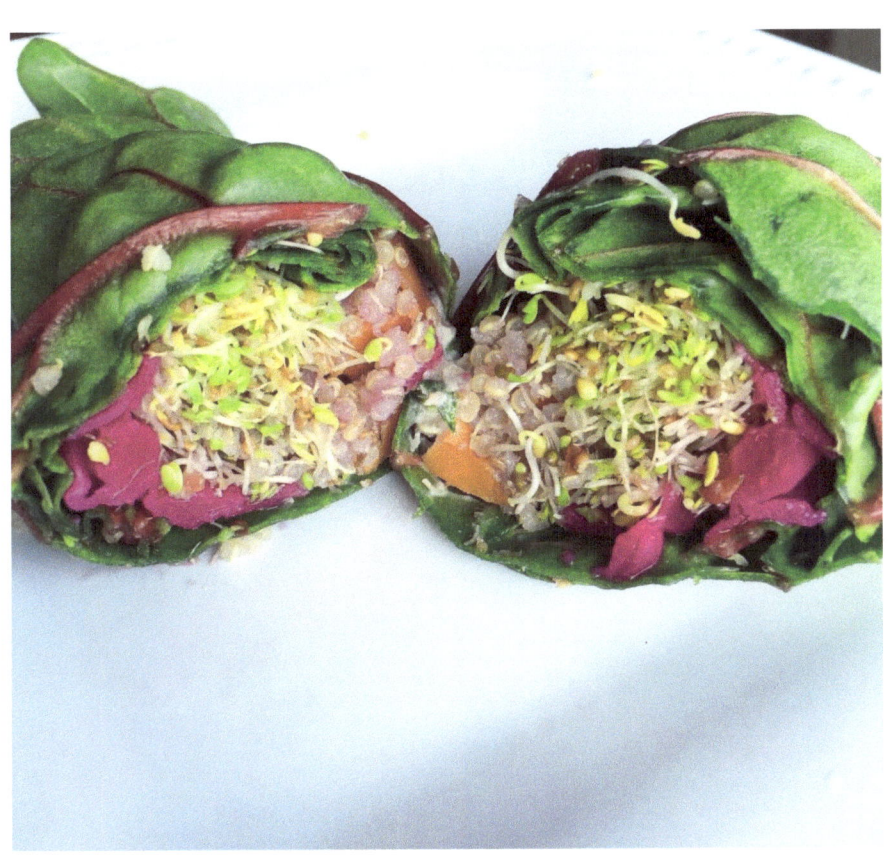

## Loaded Veggie Wrap

You can use any greens for the wrap, but in this picture I used Swiss Chard. Now just load it up with everything you have. Sprouts, cultured cabbage, quinoa, sweet potatoes, avocados, ect. You can add some kefir cheese with ranch seasoning, or simply add a little vinegar and oil to dress it up.

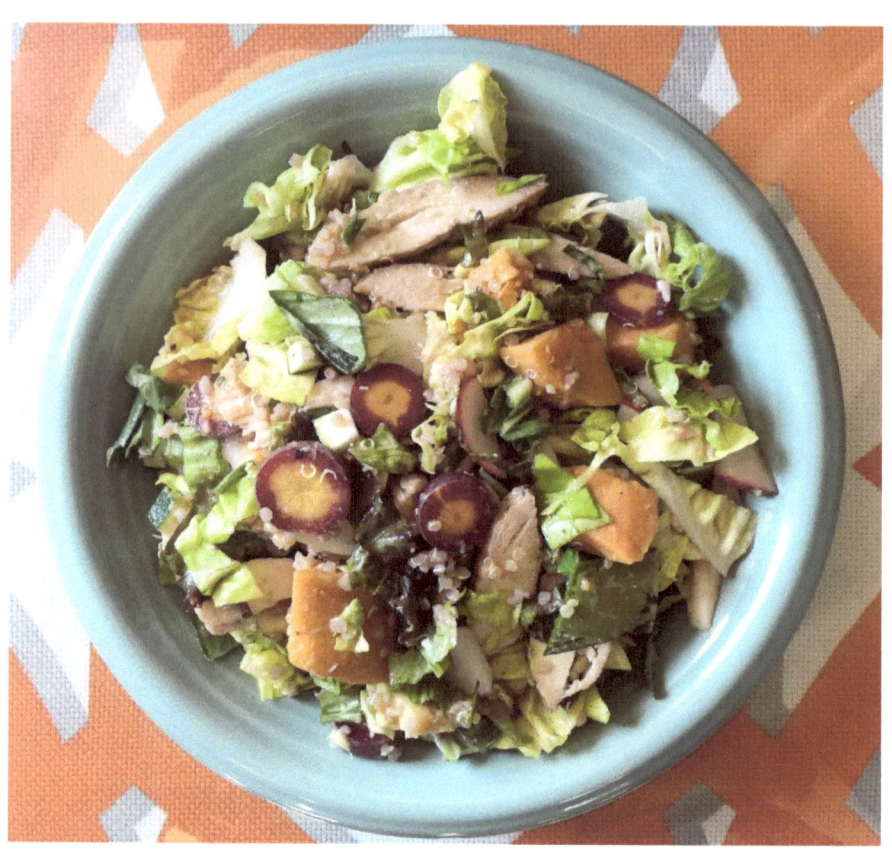

## The EVERYTHING Salad

Since we're nearing the end of the week, now it's time to use up any leftovers. I love making salads and just throwing everything in there. In this salad I have quinoa, avocados, chicken, carrots, radishes, all different greens that I had in my veggie crisper. Then for the dressing I usually use just olive oil and balsamic vinegar, with a little salt and pepper. Or I'm always in the look our for healthy dressings that don't have any sugar in them.

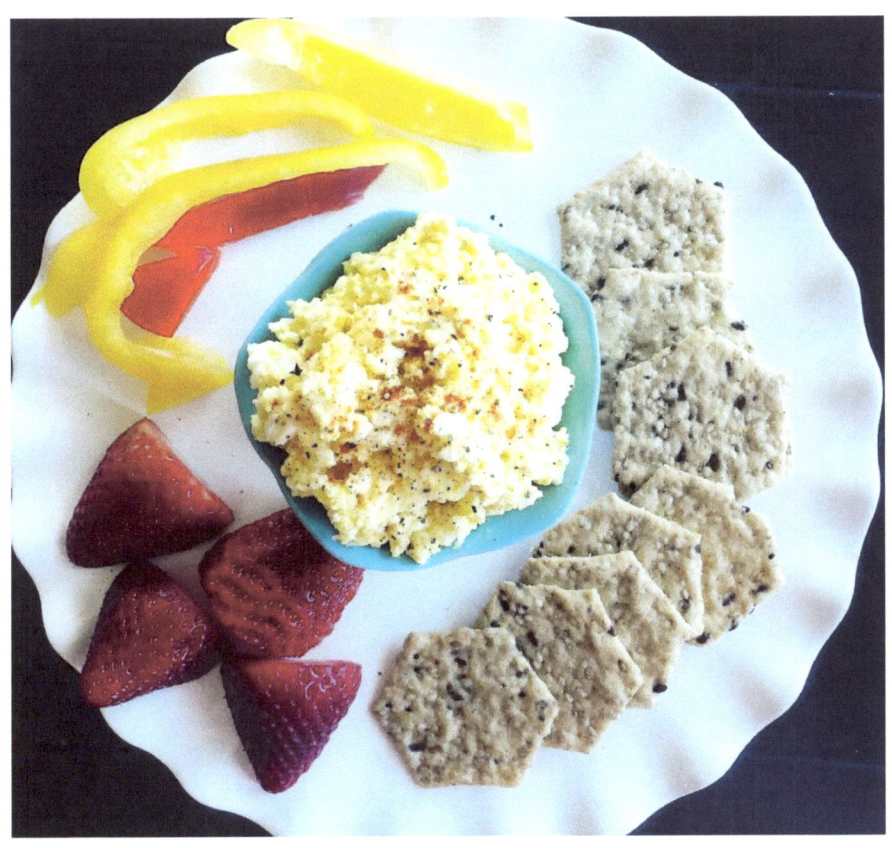

### Egg Salad w/Gluten Free Crackers

I love making big batches of egg salad, hummus or guacamole to dip my gluten free crackers in. Such and easy meal, simple yet satisfying. In this picture I just mashed up 2 hardboiled eggs, added 1 tsp. of vegan mayo (or you can use half an avocado instead of mayo), squirt of mustard, and sprinkled paprika, salt and pepper on top.

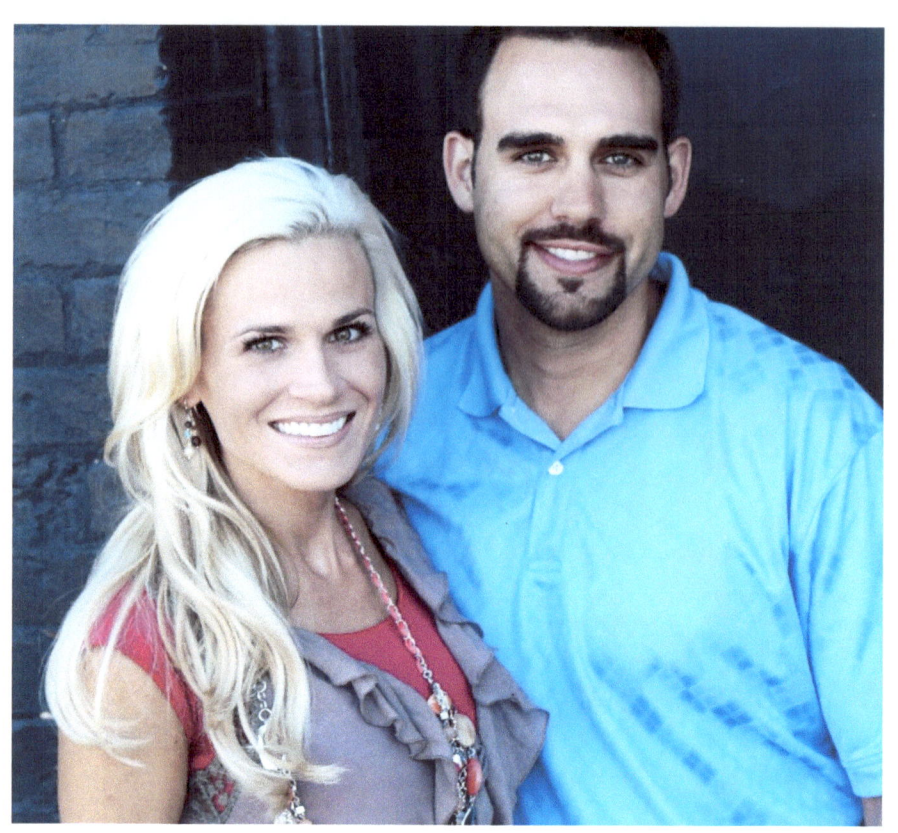

# Meet Sean & Crystal

Sean and Crystal may be the youngest Isagenix® millionaires, but their journey to success has been a long one full of lessons learned, self discovery and lots of hard work.

As the son of other Isagenix Top Income Earners, Sean knew what was possible in Isagenix. He had been taught from an early age to never work for anyone else. At age 16, his father loaned him money to start a business selling Ginsu knife sets door to door. Pretty soon, Sean started to get it; trading time for money would not create freedom and wealth.

Sean focused on developing leadership from the ground up, one person at a time. He recruited up, rather than taking the path of least resistance and enrolling everyone that looked up to him. This was especially true in the case of his most prized recruit, Crystal, who was pursuing a career with another network marketing company. Crystal's results with cleansing eventually proved to be the deciding factor in her joining Isagenix. She dropped from a size ten to a size five.* Not only did she become his business partner, but his life partner, as well.

Sean focused on developing leadership from the ground up, one person at a time. He recruited up, rather than taking the path of least resistance and enrolling everyone that looked up to him. This was especially true in the case of his most prized recruit, Crystal, who was pursuing a career with another network marketing company. Crystal's results with cleansing eventually proved to be the deciding factor in her joining Isagenix. She dropped from a size ten to a size five.* Not only did she become his business partner, but his life partner, as well.

"Joyfully overwhelmed is the only way to describe how we feel about our Isagenix success," says Crystal. "Building financial security for our posterity is what network marketing stands for." Sean adds, "It's a team effort, we owe all of our success to our mentors, but more importantly, to the beautiful people within our organization, our team!"

*We were married in July, 2004 in Salt Lake City, Utah. We have 4 children, Lily and Oliver, Brooklyn and Owen. They are truly the light of our lives. We live in our dream home in South Salt Lake Tucked away at the base of the Wasatch Mountains. During the winters we escape the freezing cold by heading south to our winter home in St. George. We've been working the Isagenix Business together since 2004 and have created Million Dollar Income by sharing this Life Transforming Nutritional Cleanse with everyone we care about. It's definitely not about the money for us, it's about what we can do with the money. More time together, less stress, the opportunity to help others and give it away. We have coached literally thousands of people through the cleansing process and the results continually blow us away every single day! We do what we love and we love what we do. We serve whom we love and we love whom we serve. "Do what you love, and you'll never work a day in your life!"*

*For individuals who dream big, are passionate about people and wish to enjoy health, rewarding relationships and financial security, Sean and Crystal Escobar are the leaders who can help you achieve personal empowerment to overcome self-limiting attitudes and realize the full power of your potential. As top leaders in the direct selling industry who love people more than they love money, Sean and Crystal have helped thousands of people discover their dreams, understand their passions and achieve their goals.*

Isagenix Introduction:

"My name is Sean Escobar, and I've been doing Isagenix for nearly 12 years now if you can believe that! Let me tell you something, for people who have tried everything out there, this is magic. My mom was the first to try it 12 years ago. She lost 14 lbs and 16 inches in just the 9 day program. She had energy to spare. My sister dropped 17 lbs and 22 inches in 9 days. My sister-in-law lost 22 lbs in 9 days. It didn't stop there. I lost 15 lbs and 15 inches in 9 days, 30 lbs in 3 weeks.. My wife shed 25 lbs and 5 dress sizes in 6 weeks. My sister Andrea dropped 100 lbs in just 5 months! (We have over 350 people who have lost over 100lbs each). It was mind blowing for all of us and that is how we became so sold on the concept of nutritional cleansing and have been sharing it with others ever since. Keep in mind that weight loss is just one benefit of this system. There are so many ancillary benefits from putting the body back in it's natural state through cleansing. It would take me much too long to write all of them, but here are just a few that people may experience: energy, mental clarity, control over cravings, healthier skin, healthier hair, stronger nails, relief from pain, motivation to get physically active, better sleep, etc.
This is not a fad diet. It is internal cleansing with the side benefit of healthy weight loss. This is not a fast, a diuretic, or colon cleanse. We do not deprive the body. It is not merely a cleanse either. It is a complete Nutritional Cleansing System that addresses all functions, facets and systems of the body at the cellular level. We do not deprive the body. We flood the body with the absolute best quality vitamins, minerals, botanicals and protein available. It's like dousing your cells with nutritional abundance unlike ever before! People love to compare things and this is generally how they establish value pertaining to a product or service. You can't compare Isagenix to anything else out there because there simply is nothing else like it in the marketplace. It is not just a shake, or simply a juice. It is a complete system. The body is a complex system, made up of many other systems. You have the digestive system, the circulatory system, the respiratory system, the elimination system, the immune system, the lymphatic system. No one nutritive or product tends to all these, it takes a system!
Isagenix is a lifestyle. In this day you simply cannot get all the necessary nutrients from the foods you eat, and our bodies are not fully able to handle the toxic burden that is placed upon them. The medical field refers to this predicament as a toxic overload or toxic body burden which may lead to different levels of auto intoxication, sometimes severe. This compromises our health on so many levels. Did you know that toxins which are not properly metabolized or eliminated get stored in fat? Google the term "toxic fat" or "toxins stored in fat." See for yourself. This form of protective fat is the most dreaded of all! You can workout till you're blue in the face and you can eat like a health nut and that stuff may not budge an inch! It won't until you properly balance your body's Ph regulatory system (ahhh yet another system!) reset, and nutritionally rebalance your body. We have seen miracles! Again, we refer to it as magic, there is simply no other way to describe it.

Isagenix is a credible company that is redefining the industry. It employs over 300 people, including 31 full time scientists. We just experienced record sales, nearly 500 million dollars in sales in our 11th year. Bottom line, results drive sales in the long run. No network marketing company can run on hype for longer than just a couple years. And there is no way my family would still be involved with the company for over a decade if the results weren't there. You might say "well the money, you stay in it for the money." Well, I welcome the money and I am grateful for it, but the money is only there because the product works. We aren't in it for the money. We have made enough money! We stay with it because it delivers for people where most everything else out there wouldn't. The commission is merely a result of our mission to help Mankind reclaim our natural birthright: our health. Our mission is to help others at this point, nothing more.

If your interest is strictly in the products then please do 2 things for me right away. #1 Go to www.isamovie.com and watch the product related videos there. #2. If you are interested in the Science behind the products then please visit www.isagenixhealth.net 3. See the Results people are experiencing. Visit www.weightlosshalloffame.net

As far as the business goes, there is no better business than Isagenix because anyone, from any walk of life, can get involved and make it BIG as a result of simply blessing other people's lives with a product that is divinely inspired in my personal opinion. I love seeing what the extra income does for people and their quality of life. It helps people begin to dream again. I would love to talk to anyone who would like to build an income source to serve their family. I can teach you how my family has earned 21 million dollars by simply sharing something that works! I'd be selfish to keep it a secret! And I genuinely believe in my heart of hearts that anyone can do it.

My father always says the following: "If you always do what you have always done, then you will always be what you have always been, and you'll always get what you've always got" -Tony Escobar. In other words, if nothing changes, nothing changes! Whether it's your health or your financial situation, if you want to see improvement, you must DO something about it.

If you are interested in the business please visit the www.isamovie.com again and watch the business videos there. Also visit www.isagenixbusiness.com to learn the compensation plan and how the business works. It is an easy business to understand and it is also a lot of fun!

If you are interested in getting started right away, please visit our personal site www.wannabelean.com and click on "sign up and save" and order one of my recommended packs there on the home page. I encourage people to try the 30 day system because there is more value there. It replaces 68 meals and comes to just around $3.50/meal. Plus it is more habit-forming, and with a 30 day money-back guarantee, there's nothing to lose, except pounds, inches and bad habits!

If you have questions, please just shoot me back an email, or you can call me at 801-979-3726. We really support our customers. In fact, network marketing was actually chosen for this product because the formulator knew it would take a personal connection and a lot of support to help people change a lifestyle. So I will coach you throughout the cleanse process. The support is the most critical factor and really helps people achieve results. This stuff flat out works!

If you are not ready to order, let's set a time to speak by phone and get any questions answered for you. Thanks for your time and I look forward to getting to know you."

~Sean